I0447414

DEVELOPING THE GRIP AND FOREARM

By

THOMAS INCH

Originally Published in 1930

PUBLISHED BY O'Faolain Patriot L L C,
Copyright 2012

info@physicalculturebooks.com

ISBN-13: 978-1475127102

ISBN-10: 1475127103

Published in the United States of America

To Order More Copies Visit:
PhysicalCultureBooks.com

1

The information contained in this publication is for historical and educational purposes only and is not designed to and does not provide medical, nutritional, or health advice, diagnosis, or opinion for any health or individual problem. The material presented is not a substitute for medical or other professional health services from a qualified health care provider who is familiar with the unique facts of the individual, and should not be used in place of a visit, call, consultation, or advice of a physician or other healthcare provider. Individuals should always consult a qualified health care provider about any health concern and prior to undertaking any new treatment. The publisher assumes no responsibility and specifically disclaims all liability for any consequence relating directly or indirectly to any action or inaction that a reader takes based on any information contained herein.

INTRODUCTION
THE GRIP IN ATHLETICS

There is a very old saying, "A chain is as strong as its weakest link".

In this connection it is rather strange how many strong men famous for their feats of strength and record breaking ability appear to fail when grip comes into play.

The author knows this is so, because of the manner in which scores of weight lifters have grumbled when they have been asked to try their strength with thick handled dumb bells, or even with a thick handled bar bell.

In the good old days when the one hand clean and jerk (or bent press) was a popular lift, it was usual to use a bent or cambered bar solely because the lifter could not go within many pounds of his limit on the lift using a straight bar through grip weakness.

Few lifters were able to pull in and jerk overhead two 56 lb. block weights, using one hand only, let alone swing them overhead. Most physical culturists have heard of the Inch Challenge Dumb Bell, the bell which defied all competitors over a very long period of years, was never lifted one inch from off the ground single handed save by the owner of the dumb bell, the author of this booklet, although the sum of £200 was offered for over 40 years and the bell made its appearance at practically every important display or weight lifting competition, also over a number of years in the Inch Strong Show upon the music halls.

Another grip test was the Inch Challenge Gripper and this has never been closed save by the owner, this refers to the latest model and not to the original grip tester which was eventually closed by Len Harvey, the famous boxer. But Harvey certainly would have little chance with the grip machine now being used in competitions and which up to the time of writing had defied many famous strong men. But the object of this introduction is to set out clearly the importance of grip in connection with many sports and games.

Take boxing, fencing, rowing, weight lifting, cricket, golf, tennis, and gymnastics. In each and every one of the foregoing it is obvious that without a good grip there will be little headway and that the better the grip the greater the success achieved. The boxer can punch harder, the fencer relies on wrist strength, grip comes strongly into rowing, the weight lifter may increase his best lifts if he can put an inch or even half an inch, upon his forearm. He will find the benefit in turning weights to the shoulder, in the two hands snatch, in dumb bell swinging and one hand snatching and, of course, in the one hand dead lift.

The cricketer relies on wrist flicks and turns in batting and bowling, this applies to the golfer in a similar manner. The tennis racquet can be swung to much better advantage when there is a grip of iron behind the movement, whilst at gymnastics there is not merely better performances with fine forearm development, but in many gym movements there is also greater safety. Body builders and weight lifters often are called upon to appear in public at a physical culture display.

Given a really good grip opportunities open up for the performer to include some simple but interesting feats such as bending iron bars, tearing packs of playing cards (Fig. 1.) or telephone books, closing a strong grip tester, raising a heavy bar bell with say a thick 1 1/2 inch bar or putting up two 56 lb. square or block weights gripped together with one hand only.

A further feat possible to the grip expert is pulling one or more men with one finger using a strap loop and here, for the benefit of those interested, it may be said that if the strap is attached to the handle of a strong expander, the opponent grasping the other handle with practise it is found that the pull of the strong rubber cords may assist the expert to succeed with his single finger pull. If a challenging strong man made an offer for any member of his audience to swing an ordinary 140 or even 150 lb. dumb bell he would soon find some takers and have to provide a medal or other reward. But if his dumb bell weighed only some 100 lbs. and had a thick handle, there is not much fear of having to part with expensive medal awards. Perhaps I have now said enough to interest the reader and lead to his working hard on lines laid down in the chapters following. I am quite sure that no one adopting the systems of grip training will regret the time given when they realise the improvement which has taken place within a very reasonable space of time.

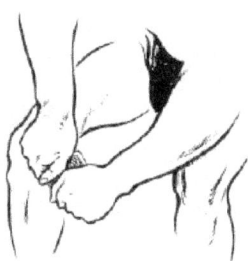

Fig. 1. Tearing a Pack of Cards

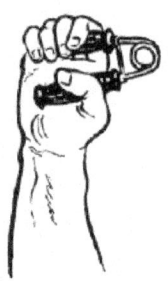

Fig. 2. Grip Tester

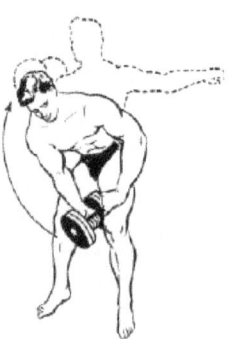

Fig. 3. Dumbbell Swing

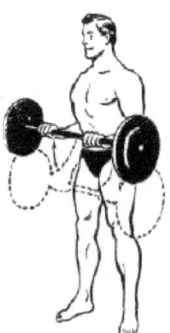

Fig. 4. Rectangular Fix

10

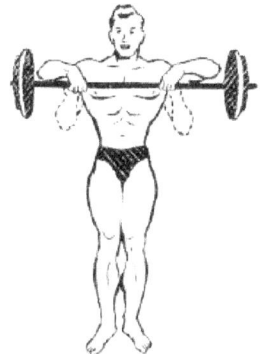

Fig. 5. Upright Rowing

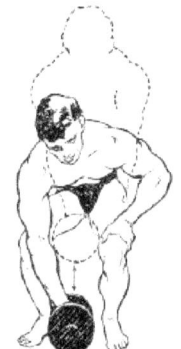

Fig. 6. One Hand Dead Lift

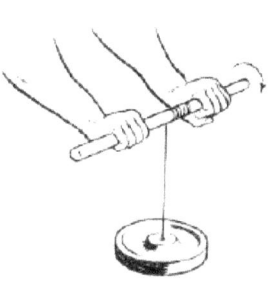

Fig. 7. Wrist Roller

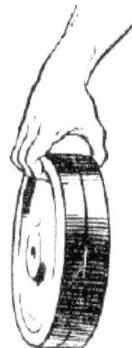

Fig. 8. Pinch Grip

Chapter 1

General Hints

Some physical culturists use chest expanders or light weight dumb bells for the purpose of home training. When this is the case there is a very simple but effective method of working which quickly improves forearm development and gives a better grip. Incidentally, it is advised that at the start of grip training the forearm is measured with the arm held out in front and straight, not bent. The forearm to be measured at its largest part and the measurement and date entered in your diary, so that a comparison may be instituted in a month or two's time. If you are possessed of a set of weights which allow a heavy barbell to be put together, then there is the test of the one hand dead lift from the floor to knee height which can also be recorded and then another test made in a couple of months time. Returning to the matter of using athletic training apparatus such as the strong expander and light dumb bells, the idea is to master a special wrist movement on the following lines and this in time will become quite mechanical yet very helpful.

Briefly, this means turning the hand and wrist as far away from yourself as possible at the start of the movement, then bringing hand and wrist over in the other direction as far as possible, giving the handle of the expander or dumb bells a good grip at the end of the movement. But taking great care NOT to keep tension or contraction on the muscles during the pull of expander or throughout the dumb bell movement. During the swing of the movement the muscles are to be relaxed and the grip only used to throw the wrist outwards at the start and inwards at the finish according to the style of exercise used. This constant flexing of the forearms and working of hand and wrist in time will give splendid results shown in better development and a noticeably better grip. Once this style is mastered then you may introduce it into your weight training. Weight training, as the average physical culturist knows, means going through a few well known lifts or movements with light weights and is not to be confused with actual heavy weight lifting. Using a comfortable weight not too heavy, you might for instance go through a few dumb bell swings and one hand snatches, a few light one hand jerks, a few presses from the shoulders and a limited number of two hand snatches, also the curl to the shoulders. In weight training one repeats the exercise a number of times without leaving go, say 5 to 10 times or whatever number you deem best. To help on grip development and at the same time assist the weight training movement you introduce the same wrist flick into the bar bell or dumb bell exercise which you did with light exercising apparatus. It is surprising when once the knack is acquired how this can help the weight lifter. No one had this down to a finer art than the late Arthur Saxon whose feats will always be famous. During his dumb bell swing on picking up he first turned the bell up with the back end down then forced the front end to go down by sheer wrist and grip power when it went between the legs before the actual swing. As it went up he gave a deliberate and forceful flick with the hand and wrist and this it may be taken added quite a good few pounds to the lift. The same thing applied when he snatched a 200 lb. bar bell single handed, a marked wrist movement flicking the bell up on its way. This movement can of course be easily applied to the two hands clean to the shoulders and the two hands snatch so that now it must be clear to the intelligent reader that besides using a special wrist movement in weight training it can also be used in actual weight lifting. One very good practise and one which should bring the idea well home to you is to load up a bar bell for the two hands clean to the shoulders. Make the bell weigh some 40 or 50 lbs. LESS than you can actually turn in when you first try this out.

When you take hold do not grip the bell tightly, do NOT close the hands. Have the hands partly open, the fingers of course crooked so that the bar lies snugly in the bent fingers. When you have taken hold in this style and as the bell starts to come up, close the hand forcibly, giving the bar a sharp flick through this closing of the hands. You will find it helps the pull in to shoulders and particularly that it is a very fine exercise referred to later on in this booklet. Once you become interested in grip training you will find it helps you in a number of ways and in due course you don't have to worry over correct procedure, you handle everything in a new style and find help from such style which onlookers fail to under stand. I have made a deep study of grip training all my life and have always found it intensely interesting and most helpful.

Chapter 2
The Grip Trainer

This little machine is most helpful for improving the tone of the forearm muscles and grip generally. I understand that the Reg Park Company supply suitable grip machines at low cost and advise each reader to obtain a pair before getting down to grip training. I myself have always used them and this has been my personal method.

Commence with the machine held in the hands at the sides of the thighs (Fig. 2). Start gripping at a fair rate of speed, not too hurriedly, and as you repeat the grips work the arms up and down slowly from thighs to shoulders. Stop a moment when the arms are bent and hands on waist level and perform several grips, then when you get to the shoulders hold them there and grip the testers till tired. If grip testers are strong then you will be compelled to make three separate sessions of the grip movements, first arms straight near thighs, then arms bent hands at waist level and finally with arms bent and the grips held near the shoulders. Generally speaking it is not necessary to count repetitions, merely continue until tired and that won't take very long I assure you. If serious business is meant the grip training system should be brought into operation twice daily, morning and evening. There is one word of warning. The tendency is for the exercises to leave the grip very tired for the time being therefore if you hit upon a weight lifting practice night it is important for you to finish with your weights before going through the grip training otherwise you would find your grip not too good for the actual lifting. Another hint worth passing on is that you thoroughly massage the tired forearm muscles after the grip training either using a little olive oil or the well known Crookes Iodine Oil.

During massage the muscles MUST be allowed to relax, never massage when they are contracted. Rub in all directions, roll and knead the muscles covering every part of the forearms opening and closing the hands whilst doing this but when you close the hands do not do 80 forcibly, avoid contracting or hardening the muscles which means you must not quite close your hands.

Chapter 3
The Thick Handled Dumb Bell

What a lot of fun I have had over many long years with thick handled dumb bells! The secret of the famous Inch Challenge Dumb Bell is of course that it has a thick handle. That and the weight of the bell has defied every famous strong man who has tried the bell and there are few who have not done so. There is no actual secret as far as the make up of the bell is concerned, the weight and the thickness of the handle call for a better grip than anyone has yet been able to exert. But it is a fact that to train with a thick handled bell helps the grip a lot and I will describe how anyone can make a thick handled dumb bell which can be used in 1) exercises, 2) the lift known as the dumb bell swing (Fig. 3), 3) the one hand clean and jerk or one hand overhead anyhow. My own bell was of course a solid bell with the weight unalterable. This would not suit the average physical culturist and so that he may use his present stock of ordinary discs, all he has to do in order to make a thick handled bell is to obtain a piece of pipe or tubing about 2 1/4 or 2 1/2 inches in diameter and about 5 inches long. Pack this by inserting other short tubes therein or using anything which fits tightly such as a pair of collars with the set screws taken out and make sure of a tight fit by packing an ordinary 1 1/8 inch steel rod with electricians tape in the centre so that there is no play of the thick tube handle. If you do not arrange a tight fit there will be bias and a dead point, the bell will not roll in the hands as it should do to make lifting difficult. Once you have succeeded as above all you have to do is load lightly for my exercises and add extra discs when you come to actual thick handle lifting. The weight used must of course suit each individual. The average physical culturist or body builder could commence with say 50 lbs. and first pull the bell from hang position between the legs several times to the shoulders first with the right hand then with the left.

In the first position the bell should be held with the palm facing inwards one set of discs to the front the other to the back. But after a rest commence again from the hang and pull the bell to the shoulder with the palm underneath and back of hand out bell longways on. Both these movements may be done till tired and of course as time goes on the weight of the bell must be slightly increased. Finally, with another one or two small discs added pull the bell to the shoulder from the floor one hand clean and jerk overhead. Endeavour to hang on to the dumb bell whilst lowering it so that it returns to the floor without the aid of the other hand. If you wish to go all out and get to your limit with the thick handle the final lift should be anyhow which means that with another one or two discs added you swing the bell unto the body and then jerk it to the shoulder by a sharp straightening of the legs and from there jerk it overhead. From time to time increase the weight and as your grip improves you will eventually be able to have fun challenging friends who visit your room or gym to raise the bell and you will find that quite a light weight dumb bell, but with a thick handle, stops them. Always try the left hand as well as the right and make sure that you fit the tube handle so that there is no dead point but a tight fit to prevent the lift being spoiled by a dead point.

Chapter 4
The Light Bar Bell

The Rectangular Fix

Years ago a popular lift was known as the rectangular fix which means standing at attention arms straight holding the bar bell near the top of the thigh. Now bring the bell up until hands are in line with the waist and hold the bell there with wrists well turned up, palms down, for two seconds to constitute a lift (Fig. 4). This is a fine movement for development of the forearm, principally the extensors. My own record at this lift was 148 lbs. The reader is advised to use a light bell from 50 to 80 lbs. as the movement should be repeated about 5 or 6 times. At the end of the repetitions you may pull the bar bell right up to the shoulders five or six times in loose easy style.

Upright Rowing

Using the same bar bell as before go through the movement known as upright rowing. Bend the arms and lean slightly forward and then work the arms exactly as in rowing (Fig. 5). After say 5 to 10 repetitions you might try reversing the movement a few times. Another very fine aid to forearm and grip development.

The Wrist Roll

Now add a substantial weight of discs to your light bell making it up to anything from 100 to 200 lbs. Pick the bell up and stand upright. Then lean slightly forward and work the bell in a wrist rolling movement which means first pulling the bell upwards towards the body with straight arms, palms inwards, bringing the bar towards the thighs by exerting your grip only. Then press it outwards as far as possible by wrist movement only. Keep this up until the forearm is definitely tired. For a change hold the bar with bent fingers, then close the hand forcibly.

The One Hand Dead Lift

If you are lucky enough to possess a good stock of discs you may now continue loading up your bell making it anything from 200 to 300 lbs. and pick up your bell single handed from the floor to above the knees (Fig. 6). Try it both left and right and after picking up with the bell longways on stand over it with the bar between the feet and pick up that style for the sake of variety. Obviously for this particular lift you must have the centre of the bell carefully marked. This one hand dead lift will act as an index showing progress.

Chapter 5
The Wrist Roll

Here is a very good forearm exercise which was a great favorite with my old friend Georges Hackenschmidt the famous champion wrestler and it may be said that Hack was almost as good with the weights as he was on the mat. Obtain a piece of wooden dowel rod about 1 1/2 to 2 inches thick and about 2 feet in length. Drill a hole through the enter of the side of the dowel. Using strong rope similar to sash line, attach 1 or 2 discs at the other end of the rope which may be about 3 feet in length. Commence with about 30 lbs. of weight and increase it as time goes on. Holding the roller waist high with bent arms and elbows well into the sides of the body, wind the discs up until they reach the wooden dowel, with your palms down (Fig. 7). Do this once or twice and then turn the hands over so that the palms are turned up.

Always continue until the forearm muscles are really tired, in all the movements like this one has to continue until there is actual pain in the muscles to get results. It may help to know that this is one of my favorite exercises and that I always use an ordinary 56 lb. block weight for this movement.

Chapter 6
The Pinch Grip

If you happen to possess some large size discs up to 50 lbs. you can try yourself out by picking one up with the finger tips and thumb (Fig. 8). Otherwise place a few ordinary ten pound discs together and after rubbing the hands and fingers with a little resin, try picking them up with one hand, and perhaps swing them out to arms length, thus exercising the deltoids as well as the grip. This kind of work definitely helps the grip.

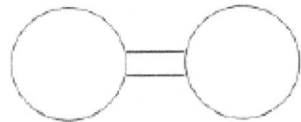

AN INTERESTING FEAT WITH THE THICK HANDLED DUMB BELL

Once the physical culturist has developed his grip until it is obviously much better than normal, he can get some fun out of setting a few feats to friends in the gym. One such feat is to load up your thick handled bell, 2 1/2 inch grip, to well over 100 lbs. and then whilst seated upon a small strong wooden box lift the bell over another dumb bell placed in front of it and then bring it back again without touching one bell with the other. At one display run at my own school in Putney some years ago and when well known lifters were present such as the well known amateur Attenborough from Derby, Aston the professional, Harold Wood, then amateur heavyweight champion of Britain, and many others, I made an offer of no less than £500 to anyone who, seated as described, could raise my challenge bell over another large dumb bell and bring it back again without their touching. It is interesting to note that I had never tried this feat before and that I was able to perform it at the first time of asking. But, of course, as no one there could move the bell when stood up, my large cash offer was perfectly safe and one or two of the lifters taking part in the display stepped forward and shook hands saying it was the finest feat they ever witnessed. At one part of this feat you appear to be holding the bell out at arms length. Needless to say, this is an optical illusion.